GASTRIC BYPASS SURGERY HANDBOOK

ALL YOU NEED TO KNOW BEFORE AND AFTER GASTRIC BYPASS SURGERY

DR. DREW NEAL

Table of Contents

CHAPTER ONE

To what extent does gastric bypass surgery work?

Obese people can benefit from the health and weight-loss benefits of gastric bypass surgery. It facilitates weight loss by reducing stomach size and altering food digestion and absorption in the stomach and small intestine. A Roux-en-Y gastric bypass is another name for this operation.

When would it be appropriate for me to consider gastric bypass?

Gastric bypass surgery may be recommended by your doctor if you are morbidly obese with other health complications despite your best efforts to shed pounds through dietary changes and increased physical activity.

Although gastric bypass surgery has been shown to be highly effective for weight loss, it is not the right choice for everyone. Talk to your doctor about your options and what to expect from treatment. You might ponder:

How much weight do people typically lose over the course of a year?

Inquiring minds want to know: • How much weight do people typically lose over the course of five years?

Inquiring minds want to know: "What am I supposed to do once I get out of surgery?"

Weight loss after gastric bypass surgery has been shown to

improve cardiovascular health, decrease the frequency of asthma attacks, and lower blood pressure.

What should I do to get ready for gastric bypass?

If you're considering surgery, you'll need to go through a battery of exams to determine whether or not a gastric bypass is safe and effective for you.

In the days or weeks leading up to surgery, your doctor will go over any necessary adjustments to your medication regimen and diet.

What exactly occurs during gastric bypass?

Having gastric bypass surgery typically necessitates 3–5 days in the hospital after administration of general anesthesia.

Keyhole surgery is the norm, but when it's not possible, open surgery is performed instead.

As can be seen in the image below, the procedure involves

the use of staples to create a small pouch in the upper portion of the stomach.

By stitching the pouch onto the lower portion of the small intestine, the majority of the stomach and the first section of the intestine are avoided.

You'll feel full on a smaller meal because less of it will be absorbed.

When I have the surgery, what should I anticipate?

After gastric bypass surgery, patients can only consume liquids for the first few weeks. After a few weeks, they'll transition to pureed food, and then solids.

After gastric bypass surgery, you'll meet with a dietitian who can give you advice on how to modify your diet for optimal health and weight loss.

And since the first part of the small intestine is responsible for absorbing a lot of vitamins and minerals, you'll have to take supplements for the rest of your life.

To successfully shed pounds, you play a pivotal role. Increasing the amount of weight you lose is possible if you stick to your diet and start moving around more. If you want to keep the weight off for good, you'll need to make these changes to your routine permanent.

What could possibly go wrong?

There is always the possibility of infection or a failed operation with any type of surgery. The staple line or the joints may leak or bleed, and bowel obstruction is always a possibility.

After surgery, low blood sugar can leave some patients feeling fatigued. Some people have trouble taking in enough food. Learn about the potential side effects of the procedure from your doctor.

Intestinal Bypass Surgery, or Roux-en-Y (RYGB)

More than 50 years have passed since the first Roux-en-Y Gastric Bypass (or simply "gastric bypass") was performed, and the laparoscopic technique has only gotten better since 1993. It's one of the most popular procedures, and it has a high success rate for curing obesity and its associated diseases. Meaning "in the shape of a Y," the name comes from the French language.

CHAPTER TWO

The Methodology

First, an upper stomach pouch (resembling the size of an egg) is created. As a result of the procedure, the larger portion of the stomach no longer stores or digests food.

Second, a new stomach pouch is created and the small intestine is divided and connected to it. It is common practice to connect the segment of small bowel that empties the bypassed or larger stomach into the small bowel some three to four feet further downstream, creating a bowel connection in the shape of the letter Y.

Third, the food will eventually be exposed to stomach acids and digestive enzymes from the first part of the small intestine that was skipped.

How It Operates

In several ways, the gastric bypass is effective. As with other bariatric procedures, the newly formed stomach pouch is smaller and has a lower capacity, resulting in a reduction in overall caloric intake. A further reduction in absorption occurs because the food does not enter the first segment of the small bowel. Importantly, altering how food travels through the digestive system has a dramatic impact on satiety, making it easier to lose weight and keep it off. Even before any weight loss occurs, the impact on hormones and metabolic health often results in improvement of adult onset diabetes. Patients with reflux (heart burn) often experience rapid symptom relief after the operation. Besides avoiding tobacco and NSAIDs like ibuprofen and naproxen, patients should also make healthy food choices.

CHAPTER THREE

1) Stable and permanent weight reduction

Remission of obesity-related conditions is achieved.

3. Method that has been perfected and standardized

Disadvantages

Surgically more involved than gastric banding or sleeve gastrectomy

Increased risk of vitamin and mineral deficiency compared to gastric banding and sleeve gastrectomy

Thirdly, there is a potential for obstruction and complications in the small intestine.

Ulcers are a potential health issue, especially for those who regularly engage in NSAID or tobacco use.

5. May lead to "dumping syndrome," characterized by nausea and/or vomiting after

consuming any type of food or drink, especially something sweet.

Anastomotic Leakage, a Complication of Gastric Bypass Surgery

Your doctor may suggest weight loss surgery if you are morbidly obese and have tried and failed to reduce your calorie intake and exercise more. Bariatric surgery is another name for weight loss surgery. In other words, it helps you lose weight and lowers your risk of health issues associated with being overweight. Some examples are hypertension, diabetes, sleep apnea, arthritis, and cardiovascular disease.

The gastric bypass is one form of surgical weight loss. Gastric bypass, like any other type of surgery, is not without its dangers. Infection, clots, and internal bleeding are all potential risks during surgery. An anastomosis is a further potential danger. The new connection between your intestines and stomach that was created during the bypass procedure will not heal properly and will cause you to develop leaks. One of the most serious risks of gastric bypass surgery is the backflow of digestive juices and undigested food through the anastomosis.

CHAPTER FOUR

Introduction to Gastric Bypass

One popular method of surgical weight loss is the gastric bypass. The upper portion of the stomach is reduced in size to create a gastric pouch during bypass surgery. The small intestine is looped, and then one end of the loop is brought up and attached to the gastric pouch. One anastomosis defines this joint. A little lower down, the remaining end of the small intestine loop is joined back up with the rest of the small intestine. Another anastomosis has been created.

You'll start feeling full sooner if you don't send your food down to your stomach first. The stomach is avoided. You won't gain weight as quickly as before because your stomach won't be digesting any of the food you eat. Afterward, you'll feel full much more quickly.

If your body mass index (BMI) is 40 or greater, or if your BMI is 35 or greater and you have severe weight-related health problems, your doctor may recommend this surgery. If your body mass index (BMI) is 40 or higher, it's safe to assume that you weigh at least 100 pounds more than you should.

Anastomotic leak symptoms

The incidence of anastomotic leaks during bypass surgery ranges from 1.5% to 6%. It could be weeks before a leak occurs. After surgery, most complication appear within the first three days. Anastomotic leak symptoms include:

An irregular or overly fast heartbeat

• Fever

Weakness in the abdomen

• Surgical incision drainage

Feeling sick to your stomach and throwing up

• Left-sided shoulder discomfort

Reduced blood pressure

Reduced urine production

Anastomotic leak risk increases with increasing obesity. In addition to being a man and having other health issues besides obesity, having a history of abdominal surgery is also a risk factor.

Treatment of anastomotic leakage and its diagnosis

Anastomotic leaking can be diagnosed with an upper GI or CT scan. Both techniques require the patient to ingest a liquid contrast dye and then undergo X-ray imaging to detect any dye loss through the anastomosis. If you experience symptoms despite a negative exam, your doctor may advise you to undergo an emergency operation to check for a leak.

In most cases, the following procedures will be carried out by the medical staff in order to treat an anastomotic leak:

• Insert an intravenous line and administer antibiotics (IV).

One option is to perform additional surgery to drain any infection caused by the leak, repair the leak, or create a new anastomosis.

• From the inside of the gastric pouch or the small intestine, place a temporary stent across the leaking area using an upper endoscopy.

The patient is to immediately discontinue all oral feedings. The leak in your intestine may be treated by being fed through a tube placed directly into the intestine.

Possibilities of Anastomotic Leakage

Bleeding and infection could occur until the leaking anastomosis is fixed. These leaks are very dangerous and could even be fatal. Ulcers, scarring, and stricturing of the anastomosis (where the intestine is connected to the gastric pouch) are possible long-term complications. Sometimes, a fistula, a skin-based drainage tube, will form. It's possible for a fistula to form connecting the gastric pouch to the remaining portion of the stomach. Because stomach acid can leak into the lungs, pneumonia is another potentially fatal complication.

Consult your doctor thoroughly before deciding to undergo gastric bypass surgery for weight loss. Consequences of obesity should be weighed against the overall risk of serious complications. Keep in mind that the best results from gastric bypass surgery can be achieved when the procedure is paired with a commitment to a long-term healthy lifestyle. The two most important of these are maintaining a healthy diet and exercising frequently.